The Essential Mediterranean Cooking Guide

Irresistible, Fit and On a Budget Recipes For Homemade Cooking

Michael Anderson

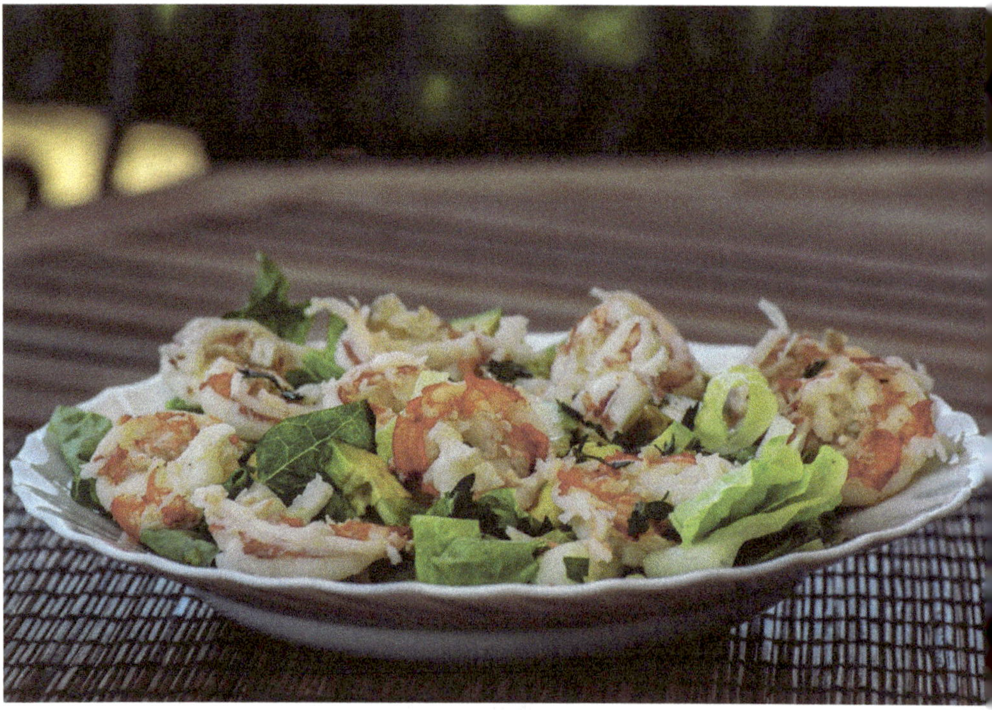

acknowledge that the author is not engaging in the rendering of legal, financial, medical or professional advice. The content within this book has been derived from various sources. Please consult a licensed professional before attempting any techniques outlined in this book.

By reading this document, the reader agrees that under no circumstances is the author responsible for any losses, direct or indirect, which are incurred as a result of the use of information contained within this document, including, but not limited to, — errors, omissions, or inaccuracies.

Table of contents

Beans, Grains, and Pastas 8
Israeli Style Eggplant and Chickpea Salad 8
Italian Sautéd Cannellini Beans 11
Lentil and Vegetable Curry Stew 12
Chickpea, Vegetable, and Fruit Stew 14
Quinoa and Chickpea Vegetable Bowls 17
Ritzy Veggie Chili 19
Spicy Italian Bean Balls with Marinara 21
Wild Rice, Celery, and Cauliflower Pilaf 24
Walnut and Ricotta Spaghetti 26
Butternut Squash, Spinach, and Cheeses Lasagna 28
Poultry and Meats 31
Panko Grilled Chicken Patties 31
Spiced Roast Chicken 33
Yogurt Chicken Breasts 35
Coconut Chicken Tenders 37
Sautéed Ground Turkey with Brown Rice 39
Baked Teriyaki Turkey Meatballs 41
Beef, Tomato, and Lentils Stew 43
Ground Beef, Tomato, and Kidney Bean Chili 44

Lamb Tagine with Couscous and Almonds 46

Chermoula Roasted Pork Tenderloin 48

Breakfast 50

Cheesy Broccoli and Mushroom Egg Casserole 50

Quinoa Breakfast Bowls 52

Warm Bulgur Breakfast Bowls with Fruits 53

Spinach Cheese Pie 55

Baked Ricotta with Honey Pears 58

Cinnamon Pistachio Smoothie 60

Breakfast Pancakes with Berry Sauce 61

Banana Corn Fritters 63

Apple-Tahini Toast 65

Marinara Poached Eggs 66

Sides, Salads, and Soups 68

Roasted Broccoli and Tomato Panzanella 68

Grilled Bell Pepper and Anchovy Antipasto 70

Marinated Mushrooms and Olives 72

Root Vegetable Roast 73

Sardines with Lemony Tomato Sauce 75

Greens, Fennel, and Pear Soup with Cashews 77

Cucumber Gazpacho 79

Veggie Slaw 80

Moroccan Lentil, Tomato, and Cauliflower Soup 82

Mushroom and Soba Noodle Soup 84

Sandwiches, Pizzas, and Wraps 86

Alfalfa Sprout and Nut Rolls 86

Mini Pork and Cucumber Lettuce Wraps 88

Mushroom and Caramelized Onion Musakhan 90

Red Pepper Coques with Pine Nuts 93

Ritzy Garden Burgers 96

Roasted Tomato Panini 99

Samosas in Potatoes 101

Spicy Black Bean and Poblano Dippers 103

Spicy Tofu Tacos with Cherry Tomato Salsa 105

Super Cheeses and Mushroom Tart 108

Beans, Grains, and Pastas

Israeli Style Eggplant and Chickpea Salad

Prep time: 5 minutes | Cook time: 20 minutes | Serves 6

2 tablespoons freshly squeezed lemon juice

1 teaspoon ground cumin

¼ teaspoon sea salt

2 tablespoons olive oil, divided

1 (1-pound / 454-g) medium globe eggplant, stem removed, cut into flat cubes (about ½ inch thick)

2 tablespoons balsamic vinegar

1 (15-ounce / 425-g) can chickpeas, drained and rinsed

¼ cup chopped mint leaves

1 cup sliced sweet onion

1 garlic clove, finely minced

1 tablespoon sesame seeds, toasted

1. Preheat the oven to 550ºF (288ºC) or the highest level of your oven or broiler. Grease a baking sheet with 1 tablespoon of olive oil.

2. Combine the balsamic vinegar, lemon juice, cumin, salt, and 1 tablespoon of olive oil in a small bowl. Stir to mix well.
3. Arrange the eggplant cubes on the baking sheet, then brush with 2 tablespoons of the balsamic vinegar mixture on both sides.
4. Broil in the preheated oven for 8 minutes or until lightly browned. Flip the cubes halfway through the cooking time.
5. Meanwhile, combine the chickpeas, mint, onion, garlic, and sesame seeds in a large serving bowl. Drizzle with remaining balsamic vinegar mixture. Stir to mix well.
6. Remove the eggplant from the oven. Allow to cool for 5 minutes, then slice them into ½-inch strips on a clean work surface.
7. Add the eggplant strips in the serving bowl, then toss to combine well before serving.

Per Serving

calories: 125 | fat: 2.9g | protein: 5.2g | carbs: 20.9g | fiber: 6.0g | sodium: 222mg

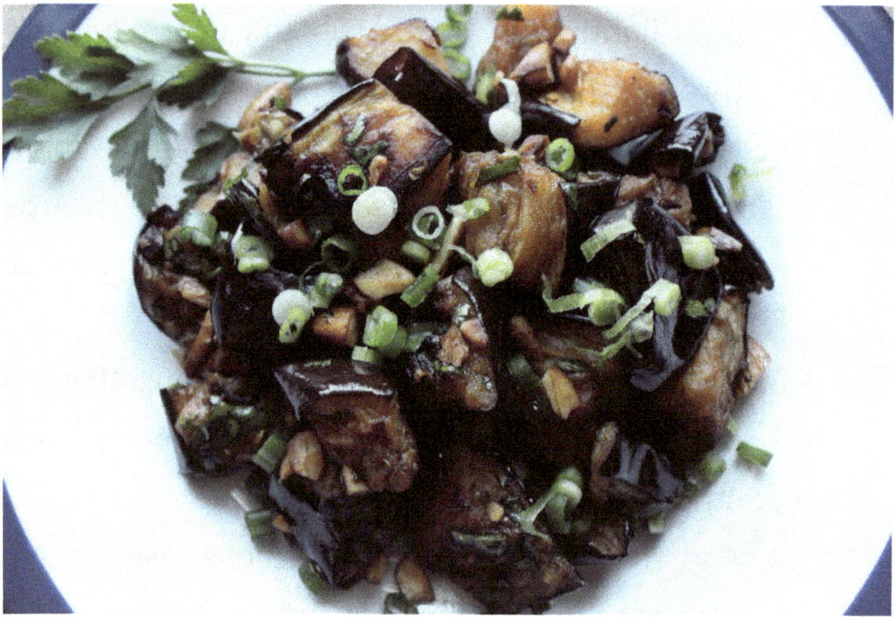

Italian Sautéd Cannellini Beans

Prep time: 10 minutes | Cook time: 15 minutes | Serves 6

2 teaspoons extra-virgin olive oil

½ cup minced onion

¼ cup red wine vinegar

1 (12-ounce / 340-g) can no-salt-added tomato paste

2 tablespoons raw honey

½ cup water

¼ teaspoon ground cinnamon

1. 2 (15-ounce / 425-g) cans cannellini beans

1. Heat the olive oil in a saucepan over medium heat until shimmering.
2. Add the onion and sauté for 5 minutes or until translucent.
3. Pour in the red wine vinegar, tomato paste, honey, and water. Sprinkle with cinnamon. Stir to mix well.
4. Reduce the heat to low, then pour all the beans into the saucepan. Cook for 10 more minutes. Stir constantly.
5. Serve immediately.

Per Serving

calories: 435 | fat: 2.1g | protein: 26.2g | carbs: 80.3g | fiber: 24.0g | sodium: 72mg

Lentil and Vegetable Curry Stew

Prep time: 20 minutes | Cook time: 4 hours 7 minutes | Serves 8

1 tablespoon coconut oil

1 yellow onion, diced

¼ cup yellow Thai curry paste

2 cups unsweetened coconut milk

2 cups dry red lentils, rinsed well and drained

3 cups bite-sized cauliflower florets

2 golden potatoes, cut into chunks

2 carrots, peeled and diced

8 cups low-sodium vegetable soup, divided

1 bunch kale, stems removed and roughly chopped

Sea salt, to taste

½ cup fresh cilantro, chopped

Pinch crushed red pepper flakes

1. Heat the coconut oil in a nonstick skillet over medium-high heat until melted.
2. Add the onion and sauté for 5 minutes or until translucent.
3. Pour in the curry paste and sauté for another 2 minutes, then fold in the coconut milk and stir

to combine well. Bring to a simmer and turn off the heat.

4. Put the lentils, cauliflower, potatoes, and carrot in the slow cooker. Pour in 6 cups of vegetable soup and the curry mixture. Stir to combine well.
5. Cover and cook on high for 4 hours or until the lentils and vegetables are soft. Stir periodically.
6. During the last 30 minutes, fold the kale in the slow cooker and pour in the remaining vegetable soup. Sprinkle with salt.
7. Pour the stew in a large serving bowl and spread the cilantro and red pepper flakes on top before serving hot.

Per Serving

calories: 530 | fat: 19.2g | protein: 20.3g | carbs: 75.2g | fiber: 15.5g | sodium: 562mg

Chickpea, Vegetable, and Fruit Stew

Prep time: 20 minutes | Cook time: 6 hours 4 minutes | Serves 6

1 large bell pepper, any color, chopped

6 ounces (170 g) green beans, trimmed and cut into bite-size pieces

3 cups canned chickpeas, rinsed and drained

1 (15-ounce / 425-g) can diced tomatoes, with the juice

1 large carrot, cut into ¼-inch rounds

2 large potatoes, peeled and cubed

1 large yellow onion, chopped

1 teaspoon grated fresh ginger

2 garlic cloves, minced

1¾ cups low-sodium vegetable soup

1 teaspoon ground cumin

1 tablespoon ground coriander

¼ teaspoon ground red pepper flakes

Sea salt and ground black pepper, to taste

8 ounces (227 g) fresh baby spinach

¼ cup diced dried figs

¼ cup diced dried apricots

1 cup plain Greek yogurt

1. Place the bell peppers, green beans, chicken peas, tomatoes and juice, carrot, potatoes, onion, ginger, and garlic in the slow cooker.
2. Pour in the vegetable soup and sprinkle with cumin, coriander, red pepper flakes, salt, and ground black pepper. Stir to mix well.
3. Put the slow cooker lid on and cook on high for 6 hours or until the vegetables are soft. Stir periodically.
4. Open the lid and fold in the spinach, figs, apricots, and yogurt. Stir to mix well.
5. Cook for 4 minutes or until the spinach is wilted. Pour them in a large serving bowl. Allow to cool for at least 20 minutes, then serve warm.

Per Serving

calories: 611 | fat: 9.0g | protein: 30.7g | carbs: 107.4g | fiber: 20.8g | sodium: 344mg

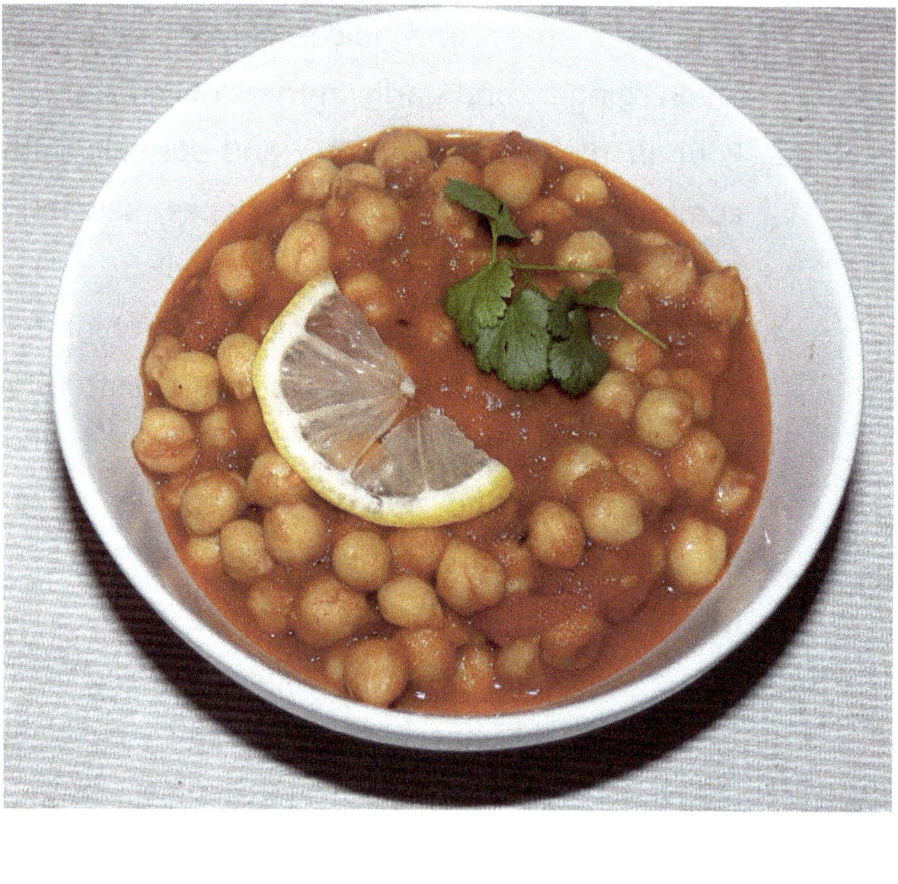

Quinoa and Chickpea Vegetable Bowls

Prep time: 20 minutes | Cook time: 15 minutes | Serves 4

1 cup red dry quinoa, rinsed and drained

2 cups low-sodium vegetable soup

2 cups fresh spinach

2 cups finely shredded red cabbage

1 (15-ounce / 425-g) can chickpeas, drained and rinsed

1 ripe avocado, thinly sliced

1 cup shredded carrots

1 red bell pepper, thinly sliced

4 tablespoons Mango Sauce

½ cup fresh cilantro, chopped

Mango Sauce:

1 mango, diced

¼ cup fresh lime juice

½ teaspoon ground turmeric

1 teaspoon finely minced fresh ginger

¼ teaspoon sea salt

Pinch of ground red pepper

1 teaspoon pure maple syrup

2 tablespoons extra-virgin olive oil

1. Pour the quinoa and vegetable soup in a saucepan. Bring to a boil. Reduce the heat to

low. Cover and cook for 15 minutes or until tender. Fluffy with a fork.

2. Meanwhile, combine the ingredients for the mango sauce in a food processor. Pulse until smooth.
3. Divide the quinoa, spinach, and cabbage into 4 serving bowls, then top with chickpeas, avocado, carrots, and bell pepper. Dress them with the mango sauce and spread with cilantro. Serve immediately.

Per Serving

calories: 366 | fat: 11.1g | protein: 15.5g | carbs: 55.6g | fiber: 17.7g | sodium: 746mg

Ritzy Veggie Chili

Prep time: 15 minutes | Cook time: 5 hours | Serves 4

1 (28-ounce / 794-g) can chopped tomatoes, with the juice

1 (15-ounce / 425-g) can black beans, drained and rinsed

1 (15-ounce / 425-g) can redly beans, drained and rinsed

1 medium green bell pepper, chopped

1 yellow onion, chopped

1 tablespoon onion powder

1 teaspoon paprika

1 teaspoon cayenne pepper

1 teaspoon garlic powder

½ teaspoon sea salt

½ teaspoon ground black pepper

1 tablespoon olive oil

1 large hass avocado, pitted, peeled, and chopped, for garnish

1. Combine all the ingredients, except for the avocado, in the slow cooker. Stir to mix well.
2. Put the slow cooker lid on and cook on high for 5 hours or until the vegetables are tender and the mixture has a thick consistency.
3. Pour the chili in a large serving bowl. Allow to cool for 30 minutes, then spread with chopped avocado and serve.

Per Serving

calories: 633 | fat: 16.3g | protein: 31.7g | carbs: 97.0g | fiber: 28.9g | sodium: 792mg

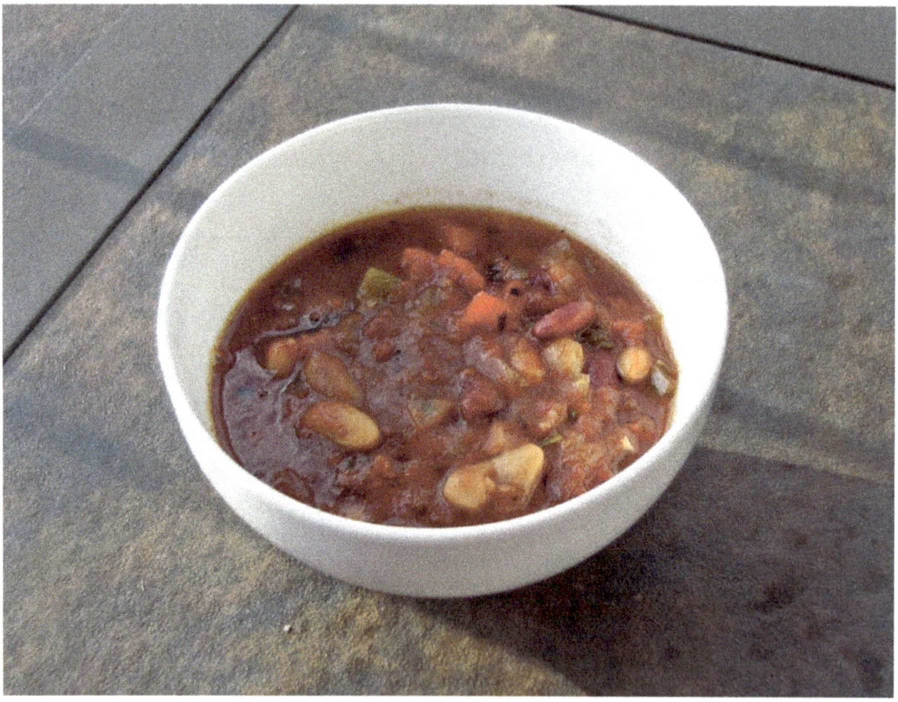

Spicy Italian Bean Balls with Marinara

Prep time: 20 minutes | Cook time: 30 minutes | Serves 2 to 4

Bean Balls:

1 tablespoon extra-virgin olive oil

½ yellow onion, minced

1 teaspoon fennel seeds

2 teaspoons dried oregano

½ teaspoon crushed red pepper flakes

1 teaspoon garlic powder

1 (15-ounce / 425-g) can white beans (cannellini or navy), drained and rinsed

½ cup whole-grain bread crumbs

Sea salt and ground black pepper, to taste

Marinara:

1 tablespoon extra-virgin olive oil

3 garlic cloves, minced

Handful basil leaves

1 (28-ounce / 794-g) can chopped tomatoes with juice reserved

Sea salt, to taste

Make the Bean Balls

1. Preheat the oven to 350°F (180°C). Line a baking sheet with parchment paper.
2. Heat the olive oil in a nonstick skillet over medium heat until shimmering.

3. Add the onion and sauté for 5 minutes or until translucent.
4. Sprinkle with fennel seeds, oregano, red pepper flakes, and garlic powder, then cook for 1 minute or until aromatic.
5. Pour the sautéed mixture in a food processor and add the beans and bread crumbs. Sprinkle with salt and ground black pepper, then pulse to combine well and the mixture holds together.
6. Shape the mixture into balls with a 2-ounce (57-g) cookie scoop, then arrange the balls on the baking sheet.
7. Bake in the preheated oven for 30 minutes or until lightly browned. Flip the balls halfway through the cooking time.

Make the Marinara

8. While baking the bean balls, heat the olive oil in a saucepan over medium-high heat until shimmering.
9. Add the garlic and basil and sauté for 2 minutes or until fragrant.
10. Fold in the tomatoes and juice. Bring to a boil. Reduce the heat to low. Put the lid on and simmer for 15 minutes. Sprinkle with salt.

11. Transfer the bean balls on a large plate and baste with marinara before serving.

Per Serving

calories: 351 | fat: 16.4g | protein: 11.5g | carbs: 42.9g | fiber: 10.3g | sodium: 377mg

Wild Rice, Celery, and Cauliflower Pilaf

Prep time: 10 minutes | Cook time: 45 minutes | Serves 4

1 tablespoon olive oil, plus more for greasing the baking dish

1 cup wild rice

2 cups low-sodium chicken broth

1 sweet onion, chopped

2 stalks celery, chopped

1 teaspoon minced garlic

2 carrots, peeled, halved lengthwise, and sliced

½ cauliflower head, cut into small florets

1 teaspoon chopped fresh thyme

Sea salt, to taste

1. Preheat the oven to 350ºF (180ºC). Line a baking sheet with parchment paper and grease with olive oil.
2. Put the wild rice in a saucepan, then pour in the chicken broth. Bring to a boil. Reduce the heat to low and simmer for 30 minutes or until the rice is plump.
3. Meanwhile, heat the remaining olive oil in an oven-proof skillet over medium-high heat until shimmering.

4. Add the onion, celery, and garlic to the skillet and sauté for 3 minutes or until the onion is translucent.
5. Add the carrots and cauliflower to the skillet and sauté for 5 minutes. Turn off the heat and set aside.
6. Pour the cooked rice in the skillet with the vegetables. Sprinkle with thyme and salt.
7. Set the skillet in the preheated oven and bake for 15 minutes or until the vegetables are soft.
8. Serve immediately.

Per Serving

calories: 214 | fat: 3.9g | protein: 7.2g | carbs: 37.9g | fiber: 5.0g | sodium: 122mg

Walnut and Ricotta Spaghetti

Prep time: 15 minutes | Cook time: 10 minutes | Serves 6

1 pound (454 g) cooked whole-wheat spaghetti

2 tablespoons extra-virgin olive oil

4 cloves garlic, minced

¾ cup walnuts, toasted and finely chopped

2 tablespoons ricotta cheese

¼ cup flat-leaf parsley, chopped

½ cup grated Parmesan cheese

Sea salt and freshly ground pepper, to taste

1. Reserve a cup of spaghetti water while cooking the spaghetti.
2. Heat the olive oil in a nonstick skillet over medium-low heat or until shimmering.
3. Add the garlic and sauté for a minute or until fragrant.
4. Pour the spaghetti water into the skillet and cook for 8 more minutes.
5. Turn off the heat and mix in the walnuts and ricotta cheese.
6. Put the cooked spaghetti on a large serving plate, then pour the walnut sauce over. Spread

with parsley and Parmesan, then sprinkle with salt and ground pepper. Toss to serve.

Per Serving

calories: 264 | fat: 16.8g | protein: 8.6g | carbs: 22.8g | fiber: 4.0g | sodium: 336mg

Butternut Squash, Spinach, and Cheeses Lasagna

Prep time: 30 minutes | Cook time: 3 hours 45 minutes | Serves 4 to 6

2 tablespoons extra-virgin olive oil, divided

1 butternut squash, halved lengthwise and deseeded

½ teaspoon sage

½ teaspoon sea salt

¼ teaspoon ground black pepper

¼ cup grated Parmesan cheese

2 cups ricotta cheese

½ cup unsweetened almond milk

5 layers whole-wheat lasagna noodles (about 12 ounces / 340 g in total)

4 ounces (113 g) fresh spinach leaves, divided

½ cup shredded part skim Mozzarella, for garnish

1. Preheat the oven to 400ºF (205ºC). Line a baking sheet with parchment paper.
2. Brush 1 tablespoon of olive oil on the cut side of the butternut squash, then place the squash on the baking sheet.

3. Bake in the preheated oven for 45 minutes or until the squash is tender.
4. Allow to cool until you can handle it, then scoop the flesh out and put the flesh in a food processor to purée.
5. Combine the puréed butternut squash flesh with sage, salt, and ground black pepper in a large bowl. Stir to mix well.
6. Combine the cheeses and milk in a separate bowl, then sprinkle with salt and pepper, to taste.
7. Grease the slow cooker with 1 tablespoon of olive oil, then add a layer of lasagna noodles to coat the bottom of the slow cooker.
8. Spread half of the squash mixture on top of the noodles, then top the squash mixture with another layer of lasagna noodles.
9. Spread half of the spinach over the noodles, then top the spinach with half of cheese mixture. Repeat with remaining 3 layers of lasagna noodles, squash mixture, spinach, and cheese mixture.

10. Top the cheese mixture with Mozzarella, then put the lid on and cook on low for 3 hours or until the lasagna noodles are al dente.
11. Serve immediately.

Per Serving

calories: 657 | fat: 37.1g | protein: 30.9g | carbs: 57.2g | fiber: 8.3g | sodium: 918mg

Poultry and Meats

Panko Grilled Chicken Patties

Prep time: 10 minutes | Cook time: 8 to 10 minutes | Serves 4

1 pound (454 g) ground chicken

3 tablespoons crumbled feta cheese

3 tablespoons finely chopped red pepper

¼ cup finely chopped red onion

3 tablespoons panko bread crumbs

1 garlic clove, minced

1 teaspoon chopped fresh oregano

¼ teaspoon salt

⅛ teaspoon freshly ground black pepper

Cooking spray

1. Mix together the ground chicken, feta cheese, red pepper, red onion, bread crumbs, garlic, oregano, salt, and black pepper in a large bowl, and stir to incorporate.
2. Divide the chicken mixture into 8 equal portions and form each portion into a patty with your hands.

3. Preheat a grill to medium-high heat and oil the grill grates with cooking spray.
4. Arrange the patties on the grill grates and grill each side for 4 to 5 minutes, or until the patties are cooked through.
5. Rest for 5 minutes before serving.

Per Serving

calories: 241 | fat: 13.5g | protein: 23.2g | carbs:6.7g | fiber: 1.1g | sodium: 321mg

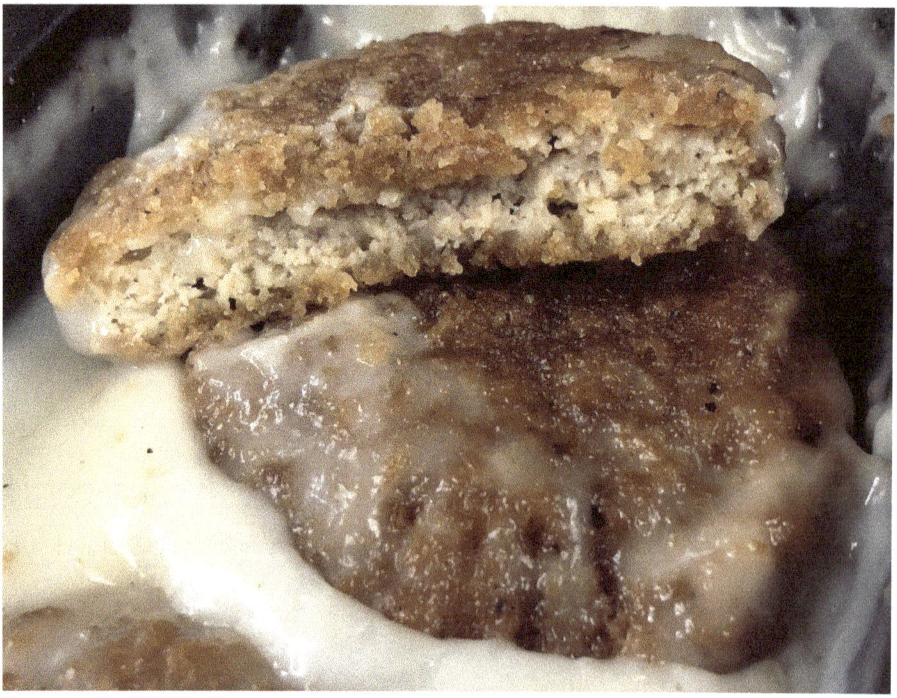

Spiced Roast Chicken

Prep time: 10 minutes | Cook time: 35 minutes | Serves 6

1 teaspoon garlic powder

1 teaspoon ground paprika

½ teaspoon ground cumin

½ teaspoon ground coriander

½ teaspoon salt

¼ teaspoon ground cayenne pepper

6 chicken legs

1 teaspoon extra-virgin olive oil

1. Preheat the oven to 400ºF (205ºC).
2. Combine the garlic powder, paprika, cumin, coriander, salt, and cayenne pepper in a small bowl.
3. On a clean work surface, rub the spices all over the chicken legs until completely coated.
4. Heat the olive oil in an ovenproof skillet over medium heat.
5. Add the chicken thighs and sear each side for 8 to 10 minutes, or until the skin is crispy and browned.
6. Transfer the skillet to the preheated oven and continue cooking for 10 to 15 minutes, or until

the juices run clear and it registers an internal temperature of 165ºF (74ºC).

7. Remove from the heat and serve on plates.

Per Serving

calories: 275 | fat: 15.6g | protein: 30.3g | carbs: 0.9g | fiber: 0g | sodium: 255mg

Yogurt Chicken Breasts

Prep time: 10 minutes | Cook time: 10 minutes | Serves 4

1 pound (454 g) boneless, skinless chicken breasts, cut into 2-inch strips
1 tablespoon extra-virgin olive oil
Yogurt Sauce:
½ cup plain Greek yogurt
2 tablespoons water
Pinch saffron (3 or 4 threads)
3 garlic cloves, minced
½ onion, chopped
2 tablespoons chopped fresh cilantro
Juice of ½ lemon
½ teaspoon salt

1. Make the yogurt sauce: Place the yogurt, water, saffron, garlic, onion, cilantro, lemon juice, and salt in a blender, and pulse until completely mixed.
2. Transfer the yogurt sauce to a large bowl, along with the chicken strips. Toss to coat well.
3. Cover with plastic wrap and marinate in the refrigerator for at least 1 hour, or up to overnight.
4. When ready to cook, heat the olive oil in a large skillet over medium heat.

5. Add the chicken strips to the skillet, discarding any excess marinade. Cook each side for 5 minutes, or until cooked through.
6. Let the chicken cool for 5 minutes before serving.

Per Serving

calories: 154 | fat: 4.8g | protein: 26.3g | carbs: 2.9g | fiber: 0g | sodium: 500mg

Coconut Chicken Tenders

Prep time: 10 minutes | Cook time: 15 to 20 minutes | Serves 6

4 chicken breasts, each cut lengthwise into 3 strips
½ teaspoon salt
¼ teaspoon freshly ground black pepper
½ cup coconut flour
2 eggs
2 tablespoons unsweetened plain almond milk
1 cup unsweetened coconut flakes

1. Preheat the oven to 400ºF (205ºC). Line a baking sheet with parchment paper.
2. On a clean work surface, season the chicken with salt and pepper.
3. In a small bowl, add the coconut flour. In a separate bowl, whisk the eggs with almond milk until smooth. Place the coconut flakes on a plate.
4. One at a time, roll the chicken strips in the coconut flour, then dredge them in the egg mixture, shaking off any excess, and finally in the coconut flakes to coat.

5. Arrange the coated chicken pieces on the baking sheet. Bake in the preheated oven for 15 to 20 minutes, flipping the chicken halfway through, or until the chicken is golden brown and cooked through.
6. Remove from the oven and serve on plates.

Per Serving

calories: 215 | fat: 12.6g | protein: 20.2g | carbs: 8.9g | fiber: 6.1g | sodium: 345mg

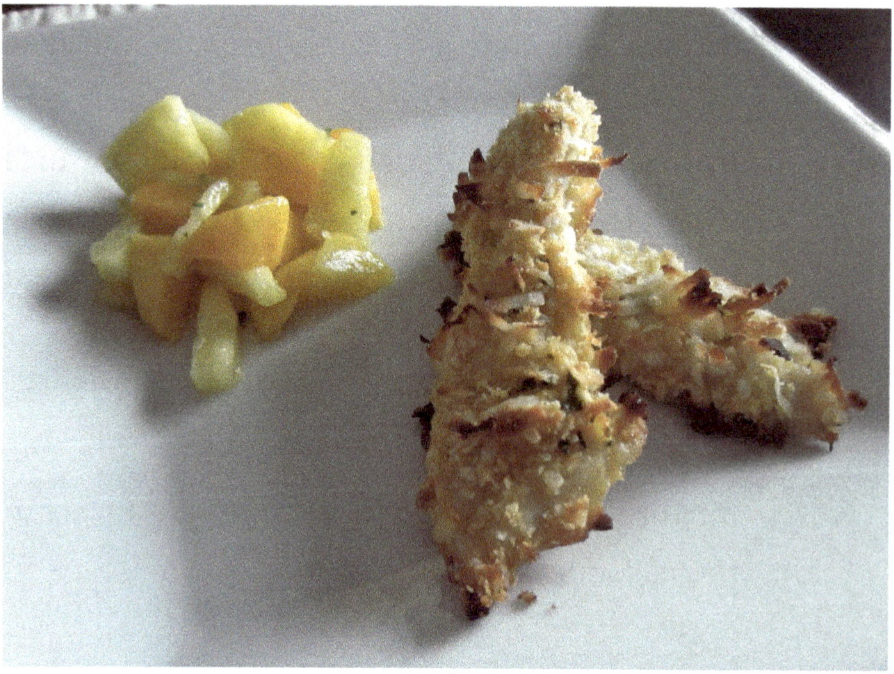

Sautéed Ground Turkey with Brown Rice

Prep time: 20 minutes | Cook time: 45 minutes | Serves 2

1 tablespoon olive oil

½ medium onion, minced

2 garlic cloves, minced

8 ounces (227 g) ground turkey breast

½ cup chopped roasted red peppers, (about 2 jarred peppers)

¼ cup sun-dried tomatoes, minced

1¼ cups low-sodium chicken stock

½ cup brown rice

1 teaspoon dried oregano Salt, to taste

2 cups lightly packed baby spinach

1. In a skillet, heat the olive oil over medium heat. Sauté the onion for 5 minutes, stirring occasionally.
2. Stir in the garlic and sauté for 30 seconds more until fragrant.
3. Add the turkey breast and cook for about 7 minutes, breaking apart with a wooden spoon, until the turkey is no longer pink.

4. Stir in the roasted red peppers, tomatoes, chicken stock, brown rice, and oregano and bring to a boil.
5. When the mixture starts to boil, cover, and reduce the heat to medium- low. Bring to a simmer until the rice is tender, stirring occasionally, about 30 minutes. Sprinkle with the salt.
6. Add the baby spinach and keep stirring until wilted.
7. Remove from the heat and serve warm.

Per Serving

calories: 445 | fat: 16.8g | protein: 30.2g | carbs: 48.9g | fiber: 5.1g | sodium: 662mg

Baked Teriyaki Turkey Meatballs

Prep time: 20 minutes | Cook time: 20 minutes | Serves 6

1 pound (454 g) lean ground turkey

1 egg, whisked

¼ cup finely chopped scallions, both white and green parts

2 garlic cloves, minced

2 tablespoons reduced-sodium tamari or gluten-free soy sauce

1 teaspoon grated fresh ginger

1 tablespoon honey

2 teaspoons mirin

1 teaspoon olive oil

1. Preheat the oven to 400ºF (205ºC). Line a baking sheet with parchment paper and set aside.
2. Mix together the ground turkey, whisked egg, scallions, garlic, tamari, ginger, honey, mirin, and olive oil in a large bowl, and stir until well blended.
3. Using a tablespoon to scoop out rounded heaps of the turkey mixture, and then roll them into balls with your hands. Transfer the balls to the prepared baking sheet.

4. Bake in the preheated oven for 20 minutes, flipping the balls with a spatula halfway through, or until the meatballs are browned and cooked through.
5. Serve warm.

Per Serving

calories: 158 | fat: 8.6g | protein: 16.2g | carbs: 4.0g | fiber: 0.2g | sodium: 269mg

Beef, Tomato, and Lentils Stew

Prep time: 10 minutes | Cook time: 10 minutes | Serves 4

1 tablespoon extra-virgin olive oil
1 pound (454 g) extra-lean ground beef
1 onion, chopped
1 (14-ounce / 397-g) can chopped tomatoes with garlic and basil, drained
1 (14-ounce / 397-g) can lentils, drained
½ teaspoon sea salt
⅛ teaspoon freshly ground black pepper

1. Heat the olive oil in a pot over medium-high heat until shimmering.
2. Add the beef and onion to the pot and sauté for 5 minutes or until the beef is lightly browned.
3. Add the remaining ingredients. Bring to a boil. Reduce the heat to medium and cook for 4 more minutes or until the lentils are tender. Keep stirring during the cooking.
4. Pour them in a large serving bowl and serve immediately.

Per Serving

calories: 460 | fat: 14.8g | protein: 44.2g | carbs: 36.9g | fiber: 17.0g | sodium: 320mg

Ground Beef, Tomato, and Kidney Bean Chili

Prep time: 10 minutes | Cook time: 15 minutes | Serves 4

1 tablespoon extra-virgin olive oil
1 pound (454 g) extra-lean ground beef
1 onion, chopped
2 (14-ounce / 397-g) cans kidney beans
2 (28-ounce / 794-g) cans chopped tomatoes, juice reserved

Chili Spice:

1 teaspoon garlic powder

1 tablespoon chili powder

½ teaspoon sea salt

1. Heat the olive oil in a pot over medium-high heat until shimmering.
2. Add the beef and onion to the pot and sauté for 5 minutes or until the beef is lightly browned and the onion is translucent.
3. Add the remaining ingredients. Bring to a boil. Reduce the heat to medium and cook for 10 more minutes. Keep stirring during the cooking.
4. Pour them in a large serving bowl and serve immediately.

Per Serving

calories: 891 | fat: 20.1g | protein: 116.3g | carbs: 62.9g | fiber: 17.0g | sodium: 561mg

Lamb Tagine with Couscous and Almonds

Prep time: 15 minutes | Cook time: 7 hours 7 minutes | Serves 6

2 tablespoons almond flour

Juice and zest of 1 navel orange

2 tablespoons extra-virgin olive oil

2 pounds (907 g) boneless lamb leg, fat trimmed and cut into 1½-inch cubes

½ cup low-sodium chicken stock

2 large white onions, chopped

1 teaspoon pumpkin pie spice

¼ teaspoon crushed saffron threads

1 teaspoon ground cumin

¼ teaspoon ground red pepper flakes

½ teaspoon sea salt

2 tablespoons raw honey

1 cup pitted dates

3 cups cooked couscous, for serving

2 tablespoons toasted slivered almonds, for serving

1. Combine the almond flour with orange juice in a large bowl. Stir until smooth, then mix in the orange zest. Set aside.

2. Heat the olive oil in a nonstick skillet over medium-high heat until shimmering.
3. Add the lamb cubes and sauté for 7 minutes or until lightly browned.
4. Pour in the flour mixture and chicken stock, then add the onions, pumpkin pie spice, saffron, cumin, ground red pepper flakes, and salt. Stir to mix well.
5. Pour them in the slow cooker. Cover and cook on low for 6 hours or until the internal temperature of the lamb reaches at least 145ºF (63ºC).
6. When the cooking is complete, mix in the honey and dates, then cook for another an hour.
7. Put the couscous in a tagine bowl or a large bowl, then top with lamb mixture. Scatter with slivered almonds and serve immediately.

Per Serving

calories: 447 | fat: 10.2g | protein: 36.3g | carbs: 53.5g | fiber: 4.9g | sodium: 329mg

Chermoula Roasted Pork Tenderloin

Prep time: 15 minutes | Cook time: 20 minutes | Serves 2

½ cup fresh cilantro
½ cup fresh parsley
6 small garlic cloves
3 tablespoons olive oil, divided
3 tablespoons freshly squeezed lemon juice
2 teaspoons cumin
1 teaspoon smoked paprika
½ teaspoon salt, divided
Pinch freshly ground black pepper
1 (8-ounce / 227-g) pork tenderloin

1. Preheat the oven to 425ºF (220ºC).
2. In a food processor, combine the cilantro, parsley, garlic, 2 tablespoons of olive oil, lemon juice, cumin, paprika, and ¼ teaspoon of salt. Pulse 15 to 20 times, or until the mixture is fairly smooth. Scrape the sides down as needed to incorporate all the ingredients. Transfer the sauce to a small bowl and set aside.
3. Season the pork tenderloin on all sides with the remaining ¼ teaspoon of salt and a generous pinch of black pepper.

4. Heat the remaining 1 tablespoon of olive oil in a sauté pan.
5. Sear the pork for 3 minutes, turning often, until golden brown on all sides.
6. Transfer the pork to a baking dish and roast in the preheated oven for 15 minutes, or until the internal temperature registers 145ºF (63ºC).
7. Cool for 5 minutes before serving.

Per Serving

calories: 169 | fat: 13.1g | protein: 11.0g | carbs: 2.9g | fiber: 1.0g | sodium: 332mg

Breakfast

Cheesy Broccoli and Mushroom Egg Casserole

Prep time: 10 minutes | Cook time: 40 minutes | Serves 4

2 tablespoons extra-virgin olive oil

½ sweet onion, chopped

1 teaspoon minced garlic

1 cup sliced button mushrooms

1 cup chopped broccoli

8 large eggs

¼ cup unsweetened almond milk

1 tablespoon chopped fresh basil

1 cup shredded Cheddar cheese

Sea salt and freshly ground black pepper, to taste

1. Preheat the oven to 375ºF (190ºC).
2. Heat the olive oil in a large ovenproof skillet over medium-high heat.
3. Add the onion, garlic, and mushrooms to the skillet and sauté for about 5 minutes, stirring occasionally.

4. Stir in the broccoli and sauté for 5 minutes until the vegetables start to soften.
5. Meanwhile, beat the eggs with the almond milk and basil in a small bowl until well mixed.
6. Remove the skillet from the heat and pour the egg mixture over the top. Scatter the Cheddar cheese all over.
7. Bake uncovered in the preheated oven for about 30 minutes, or until the top of the casserole is golden brown and a fork inserted in the center comes out clean.
8. Remove from the oven and sprinkle with the sea salt and pepper. Serve hot.

Per Serving

calories: 326 | fat: 27.2g | protein: 14.1g | carbs: 6.7g | fiber: 0.7g | sodium: 246mg

Quinoa Breakfast Bowls

Prep time: 5 minutes | Cook time: 17 minutes | Serves 1

¼ cup quinoa, rinsed

¾ cup water, plus additional as needed

1 carrot, grated

½ small broccoli head, finely chopped

¼ teaspoon salt

1 tablespoon chopped fresh dill

1. Add the quinoa and water to a small pot over high heat and bring to a boil.
2. Once boiling, reduce the heat to low. Cover and cook for 5 minutes, stirring occasionally.
3. Stir in the carrot, broccoli, and salt and continue cooking for 1o to 12 minutes, or until the quinoa is cooked though and the vegetables are fork- tender. If the mixture gets too thick, you can add additional water as needed.
4. Add the dill and serve warm.

Per Serving

calories: 219 | fat: 2.9g | protein: 10.0g | carbs: 40.8g | fiber: 7.1g | sodium: 666mg

Warm Bulgur Breakfast Bowls with Fruits

Prep time: 5 minutes | Cook time: 15 minutes | Serves 6

2 cups unsweetened almond milk

1½ cups uncooked bulgur

1 cup water

½ teaspoon ground cinnamon

2 cups frozen (or fresh, pitted) dark sweet cherries

8 dried (or fresh) figs, chopped

½ cup chopped almonds

¼ cup loosely packed fresh mint, chopped

1. Combine the milk, bulgur, water, and cinnamon in a medium saucepan, stirring, and bring just to a boil.
2. Cover, reduce the heat to medium-low, and allow to simmer for 10 minutes, or until the liquid is absorbed.
3. Turn off the heat, but keep the pan on the stove, and stir in the frozen cherries (no need to thaw), figs, and almonds. Cover and let the hot bulgur thaw the cherries and partially hydrate the figs, about 1 minute.
4. Fold in the mint and stir to combine, then serve.

Per Serving

calories: 207 | fat: 6.0g | protein: 8.0g | carbs: 32.0g | fiber: 4.0g | sodium: 82mg

Spinach Cheese Pie

Prep time: 5 minutes | Cook time: 25 minutes | Serves 8

2 tablespoons extra-virgin olive oil

1 onion, chopped

1 pound (454 g) frozen spinach, thawed

¼ teaspoon ground nutmeg

¼ teaspoon garlic salt

¼ teaspoon freshly ground black pepper

4 large eggs, divided

1 cup grated Parmesan cheese, divided

2 puff pastry doughs, at room temperature

4 hard-boiled eggs, halved

Nonstick cooking spray

1. Preheat the oven to 350ºF (180ºC). Spritz a baking sheet with nonstick cooking spray and set aside.
2. Heat a large skillet over medium-high heat. Add the olive oil and onion and sauté for about 5 minutes, stirring occasionally, or until translucent.
3. Squeeze the excess water from the spinach, then add to the skillet and cook, uncovered, so

that any excess water from the spinach can evaporate.

4. Season with the nutmeg, garlic salt, and black pepper. Remove from heat and set aside to cool.
5. Beat 3 eggs in a small bowl. Add the beaten eggs and ½ cup of Parmesan cheese to the spinach mixture, stirring well.
6. Roll out the pastry dough on the prepared baking sheet. Layer the spinach mixture on top of the dough, leaving 2 inches around each edge.
7. Once the spinach is spread onto the pastry dough, evenly place the hard-boiled egg halves throughout the pie, then cover with the second pastry dough. Pinch the edges closed.
8. Beat the remaining 1 egg in the bowl. Brush the egg wash over the pastry dough.
9. Bake in the preheated oven for 15 to 20 minutes until golden brown.
10. Sprinkle with the remaining ½ cup of Parmesan cheese. Cool for 5 minutes before cutting and serving.

Per Serving

calories: 417 | fat: 28.0g | protein: 17.0g | carbs: 25.0g | fiber: 3.0g | sodium: 490mg

Baked Ricotta with Honey Pears

Prep time: 5 minutes | Cook time: 22 to 25 minutes | Serves 4

1 (1-pound / 454-g) container whole-milk ricotta cheese

2 large eggs

¼ cup whole-wheat pastry flour

1 tablespoon sugar

1 teaspoon vanilla extract

¼ teaspoon ground nutmeg

1 pear, cored and diced

2 tablespoons water

1 tablespoon honey

Nonstick cooking spray

1. Preheat the oven to 400ºF (205ºC). Spray four ramekins with nonstick cooking spray.
2. Beat together the ricotta, eggs, flour, sugar, vanilla, and nutmeg in a large bowl until combined. Spoon the mixture into the ramekins.
3. Bake in the preheated oven for 22 to 25 minutes, or until the ricotta is just set.
4. Meanwhile, in a small saucepan over medium heat, simmer the pear in the water for 10 minutes, or until slightly softened. Remove from the heat, and stir in the honey.

5. Remove the ramekins from the oven and cool slightly on a wire rack. Top the ricotta ramekins with the pear and serve.

Per Serving

calories: 329 | fat: 19.0g | protein: 17.0g | carbs: 23.0g | fiber: 3.0g | sodium: 109mg

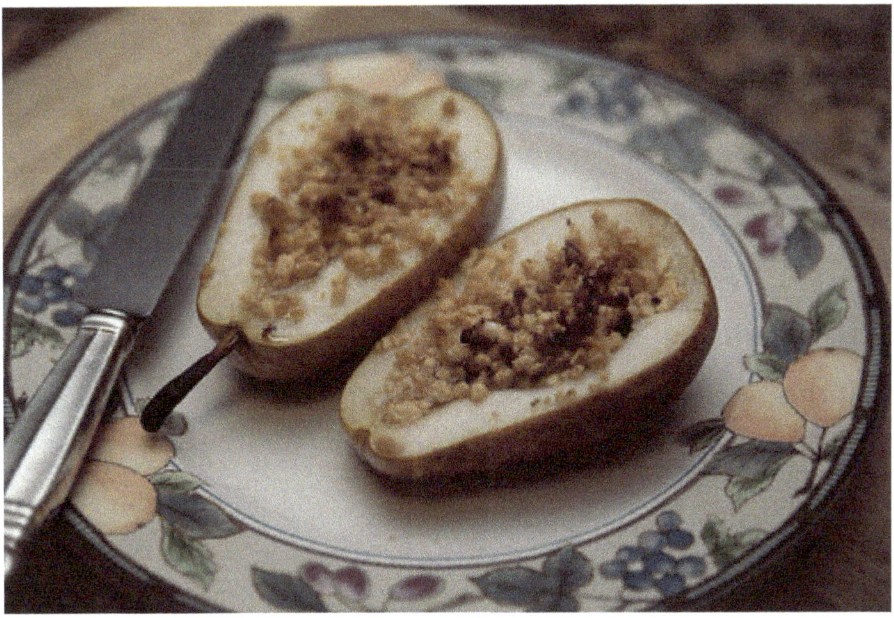

Cinnamon Pistachio Smoothie

Prep time: 5 minutes | Cook time: 0 minutes | Serves 1

½ cup unsweetened almond milk, plus more as needed

½ cup plain Greek yogurt

Zest and juice of ½ orange

1 tablespoon extra-virgin olive oil

1 tablespoon shelled pistachios, coarsely chopped

¼ to ½ teaspoon ground allspice

¼ teaspoon vanilla extract

¼ teaspoon ground cinnamon

1. In a blender, combine ½ cup almond milk, yogurt, orange zest and juice, olive oil, pistachios, allspice, vanilla, and cinnamon. Blend until smooth and creamy, adding more almond milk to achieve your desired consistency.
2. Serve chilled.

Per Serving

calories: 264 | fat: 22.0g | protein: 6.0g | carbs: 12.0g | fiber: 2.0g | sodium: 127mg

Breakfast Pancakes with Berry Sauce

Prep time: 5 minutes | Cook time: 10 minutes | Serves 4

Pancakes:

1 cup almond flour

1 teaspoon baking powder

¼ teaspoon salt

6 tablespoon extra-virgin olive oil, divided

2 large eggs, beaten

Zest and juice of 1 lemon

½ teaspoon vanilla extract

Berry Sauce:

1 cup frozen mixed berries

1 tablespoon water, plus more as needed

½ teaspoon vanilla extract

Make the Pancakes

1. In a large bowl, combine the almond flour, baking powder, and salt and stir to break up any clumps.
2. Add 4 tablespoons olive oil, beaten eggs, lemon zest and juice, and vanilla extract and stir until well mixed.
3. Heat 1 tablespoon of olive oil in a large skillet. Spoon about 2 tablespoons of batter for each pancake. Cook until bubbles begin to form, 4 to 5 minutes. Flip and cook for another 2 to 3

minutes. Repeat with the remaining 1 tablespoon of olive oil and batter.

Make the Berry Sauce

4. Combine the frozen berries, water, and vanilla extract in a small saucepan and heat over medium-high heat for 3 to 4 minutes until bubbly, adding more water as needed. Using the back of a spoon or fork, mash the berries and whisk until smooth.
5. Serve the pancakes with the berry sauce.

Per Serving

calories: 275 | fat: 26.0g | protein: 4.0g | carbs: 8.0g | fiber: 2.0g | sodium: 271mg

Banana Corn Fritters

Prep time: 5 minutes | Cook time: 10 minutes | Serves 2

½ cup yellow cornmeal

¼ cup flour

2 small ripe bananas, peeled and mashed

2 tablespoons unsweetened almond milk

1 large egg, beaten

½ teaspoon baking powder

¼ to ½ teaspoon ground chipotle chili

¼ teaspoon ground cinnamon

¼ teaspoon sea salt

1 tablespoon olive oil

1. Stir together all ingredients except for the olive oil in a large bowl until smooth.
2. Heat a nonstick skillet over medium-high heat. Add the olive oil and drop about 2 tablespoons of batter for each fritter. Cook for 2 to 3 minutes until the bottoms are golden brown, then flip. Continue cooking for 1 to 2 minutes more, until cooked through. Repeat with the remaining batter.
3. Serve warm.

Per Serving

calories: 396 | fat: 10.6g | protein: 7.3g | carbs: 68.0g | fiber: 4.8g | sodium: 307mg

Apple-Tahini Toast

Prep time: 5 minutes | Cook time: 0 minutes | Serves 1

2 slices whole-wheat bread, toasted

2 tablespoons tahini

1 small apple of your choice, cored and thinly sliced

1 teaspoon honey

1. Spread the tahini on the toasted bread.
2. Place the apple slices on the bread and drizzle with the honey. Serve immediately.

Per Serving

calories: 458 | fat: 17.8g | protein: 11.0g | carbs: 63.5g | fiber: 10.5g | sodium: 285mg

Marinara Poached Eggs

Prep time: 5 minutes | Cook time: 15 minutes | Serves 6

1 tablespoon extra-virgin olive oil

1 cup chopped onion

2 garlic cloves, minced

2 (14.5-ounce / 411-g) cans no-salt-added Italian diced tomatoes, undrained

6 large eggs

½ cup chopped fresh flat-leaf parsley

1. Heat the olive oil in a large skillet over medium-high heat.
2. Add the onion and sauté for 5 minutes, stirring occasionally. Add the garlic and cook for 1 minute more.
3. Pour the tomatoes with their juices over the onion mixture and cook for 2 to 3 minutes until bubbling.
4. Reduce the heat to medium and use a large spoon to make six indentations in the tomato mixture. Crack the eggs, one at a time, into each indentation.
5. Cover and simmer for 6 to 7 minutes, or until the eggs are cooked to your preference.

6. Serve with the parsley sprinkled on top.

Per Serving

calories: 89 | fat: 6.0g | protein: 4.0g | carbs: 4.0g | fiber: 1.0g | sodium: 77mg

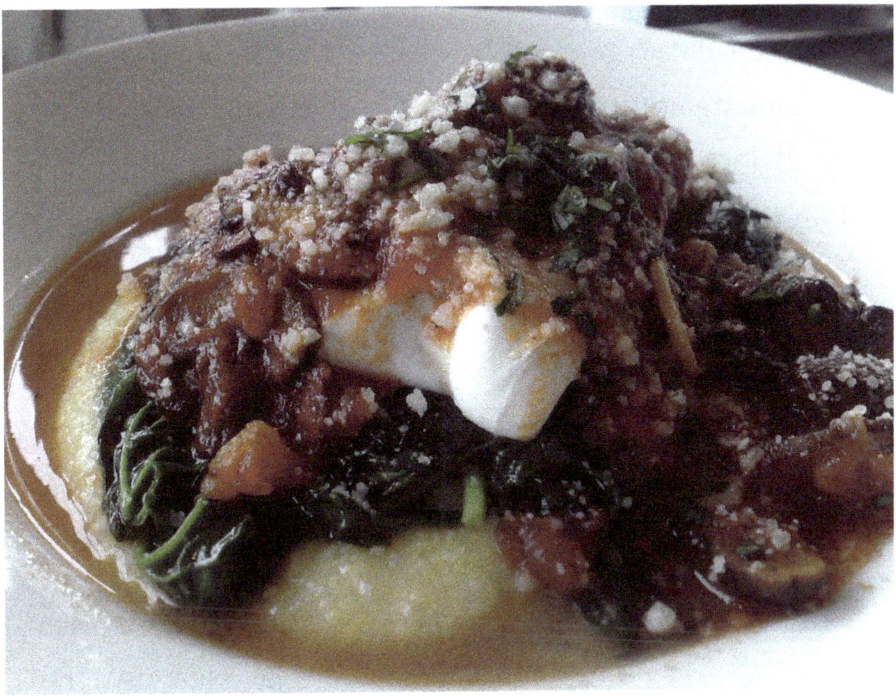

Sides, Salads, and Soups

Roasted Broccoli and Tomato Panzanella

Prep time: 10 minutes | Cook time: 20 minutes | Serves 4

1 pound (454 g) broccoli (about 3 medium stalks), trimmed, cut into 1- inch florets and ½-inch stem slices

2 tablespoons extra-virgin olive oil, divided

1½ cups cherry tomatoes

1½ teaspoons honey, divided

3 cups cubed whole-grain crusty bread

1 tablespoon balsamic vinegar

¼ teaspoon kosher salt

½ teaspoon freshly ground black pepper

¼ cup grated Parmesan cheese, for serving (optional)

¼ cup chopped fresh oregano leaves, for serving (optional)

1. Preheat the oven to 450ºF (235ºC).
2. Toss the broccoli with 1 tablespoon of olive oil in a large bowl to coat well.
3. Arrange the broccoli on a baking sheet, then add the tomatoes to the same bowl and toss

with the remaining olive oil. Add 1 teaspoon of honey and toss again to coat well. Transfer the tomatoes on the baking sheet beside the broccoli.

4. Place the baking sheet in the preheated oven and roast for 15 minutes, then add the bread cubes and flip the vegetables. Roast for an additional 3 minutes or until the broccoli is lightly charred and the bread cubes are golden brown.
5. Meanwhile, combine the remaining ingredients, except for the Parmesan and oregano, in a small bowl. Stir to mix well.
6. Transfer the roasted vegetables and bread cubes to the large salad bowl, then dress them and spread with Parmesan and oregano leaves. Toss and serve immediately.

Per Serving

calories: 162 | fat: 6.8g | protein: 8.2g | carbs: 18.9g | fiber: 6.0g | sodium: 397mg

Grilled Bell Pepper and Anchovy Antipasto

Prep time: 15 minutes | Cook time: 8 minutes | Serves 4

2 tablespoons extra-virgin olive oil, divided

4 medium red bell peppers, quartered, stem and seeds removed

6 ounces (170 g) anchovies in oil, chopped

2 tablespoons capers, rinsed and drained

1 cup Kalamata olives, pitted

1 small shallot, chopped

Sea salt and freshly ground pepper, to taste

1. Heat the grill to medium-high heat. Grease the grill grates with 1 tablespoon of olive oil.
2. Arrange the red bell peppers on the preheated grill grates, then grill for 8 minutes or until charred.
3. Turn off the grill and allow the pepper to cool for 10 minutes.
4. Transfer the charred pepper in a colander. Rinse and peel the peppers under running cold water, then pat dry with paper towels.

5. Cut the peppers into chunks and combine with remaining ingredients in a large bowl. Toss to mix well.
6. Serve immediately.

Per Serving

calories: 227 | fat: 14.9g | protein: 13.9g | carbs: 9.9g | fiber: 3.8g| sodium: 1913mg

Marinated Mushrooms and Olives

Prep time: 1 hour 10 minutes | Cook time: 0 minutes | Serves 8

- 1 pound (454 g) white button mushrooms, rinsed and drained
- 1 pound (454 g) fresh olives
- ½ tablespoon crushed fennel seeds
- 1 tablespoon white wine vinegar
- 2 tablespoons fresh thyme leaves
- Pinch chili flakes
- Sea salt and freshly ground pepper, to taste
- 2 tablespoons extra-virgin olive oil

1. Combine all the ingredients in a large bowl. Toss to mix well.
2. Wrap the bowl in plastic and refrigerate for at least 1 hour to marinate.
3. Remove the bowl from the refrigerate and let sit under room temperature for 10 minutes, then serve.

Per Serving

calories: 111 | fat: 9.7g | protein: 2.4g | carbs: 5.9g | fiber: 2.7g | sodium: 449mg

Root Vegetable Roast

Prep time: 15 minutes | Cook time: 25 minutes | Serves 4 to 6

1 bunch beets, peeled and cut into 1-inch cubes

2 small sweet potatoes, peeled and cut into 1-inch cubes

3 parsnips, peeled and cut into 1-inch rounds

4 carrots, peeled and cut into 1-inch rounds

1 tablespoon raw honey

1 teaspoon sea salt

½ teaspoon freshly ground black pepper

1 tablespoon extra-virgin olive oil

2 tablespoons coconut oil, melted

1. Preheat the oven to 400ºF (205ºC). Line a baking sheet with parchment paper.
2. Combine all the ingredients in a large bowl. Toss to coat the vegetables well.
3. Pour the mixture in the baking sheet, then place the sheet in the preheated oven.
4. Roast for 25 minutes or until the vegetables are lightly browned and soft. Flip the vegetables halfway through the cooking time.
5. Remove the vegetables from the oven and allow to cool before serving.

Per Serving

calories: 461 | fat: 18.1g | protein: 5.9g | carbs: 74.2g | fiber: 14.0g | sodium: 759mg

Sardines with Lemony Tomato Sauce

Prep time: 10 minutes | Cook time: 40 minutes | Serves 4

2 tablespoons olive oil, divided

4 Roma tomatoes, peeled and chopped, reserve the juice

1 small onion, sliced thinly

Zest of 1 orange

Sea salt and freshly ground pepper, to taste

1 pound (454 g) fresh sardines, rinsed, spine removed, butterflied

½ cup white wine

2 tablespoons whole-wheat breadcrumbs

1. Preheat the oven to 425ºF (220ºC). Grease a baking dish with 1 tablespoon of olive oil.
2. Heath the remaining olive oil in a nonstick skillet over medium-low heat until shimmering.
3. Add the tomatoes with juice, onion, orange zest, salt, and ground pepper to the skillet and simmer for 20 minutes or until it thickens.
4. Pour half of the mixture on the bottom of the baking dish, then top with the butterflied

sardines. Pour the remaining mixture and white wine over the sardines.

5. Spread the breadcrumbs on top, then place the baking dish in the preheated oven. Bake for 20 minutes or until the fish is opaque.
6. Remove the baking sheet from the oven and serve the sardines warm.

Per Serving

calories: 363 | fat: 20.2g | protein: 29.7g | carbs: 9.7g | fiber: 2.0g| sodium: 381mg

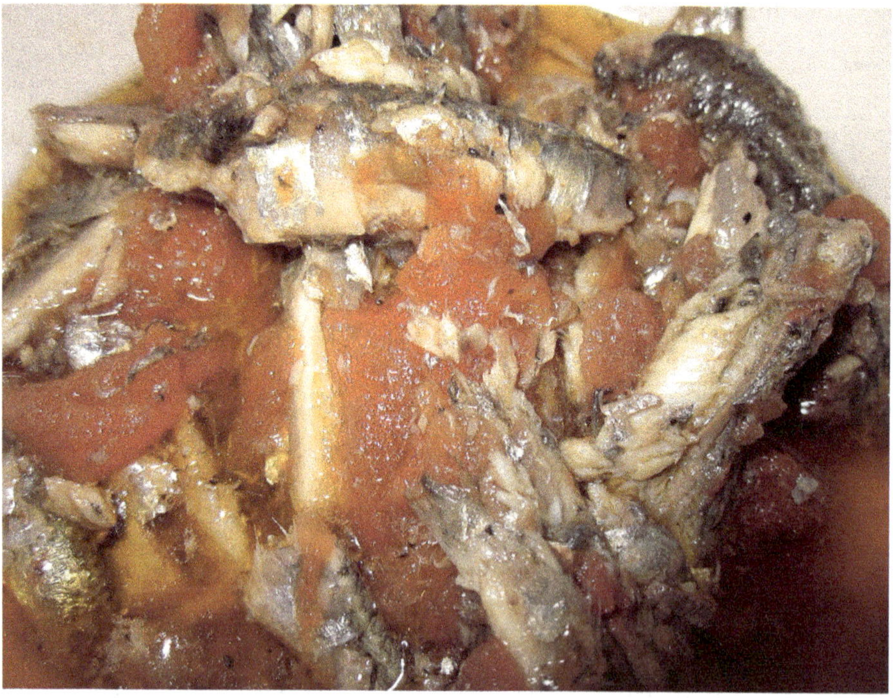

Greens, Fennel, and Pear Soup with Cashews

Prep time: 15 minutes | Cook time: 15 minutes | Serves 4 to 6

2 tablespoons olive oil

1 fennel bulb, cut into ¼-inch-thick slices

2 leeks, white part only, sliced

2 pears, peeled, cored, and cut into ½-inch cubes

1 teaspoon sea salt

¼ teaspoon freshly ground black pepper

½ cup cashews

2 cups packed blanched spinach

3 cups low-sodium vegetable soup

1. Heat the olive oil in a stockpot over high heat until shimmering.
2. Add the fennel and leeks, then sauté for 5 minutes or until tender.
3. Add the pears and sprinkle with salt and pepper, then sauté for another 3 minutes or until the pears are soft.
4. Add the cashews, spinach, and vegetable soup. Bring to a boil. Reduce the heat to low. Cover and simmer for 5 minutes.

5. Pour the soup in a food processor, then pulse until creamy and smooth.
6. Pour the soup back to the pot and heat over low heat until heated through.
7. Transfer the soup to a large serving bowl and serve immediately.

Per Serving

calories: 266 | fat: 15.1g | protein: 5.2g | carbs: 32.9g | fiber: 7.0g | sodium: 628mg

Cucumber Gazpacho

Prep time: 10 minutes | Cook time: 0 minutes | Serves 4

- 2 cucumbers, peeled, deseeded, and cut into chunks
- ½ cup mint, finely chopped
- 2 cups plain Greek yogurt
- 2 garlic cloves, minced
- 2 cups low-sodium vegetable soup
- 1 tablespoon no-salt-added tomato paste
- 3 teaspoons fresh dill
- Sea salt and freshly ground pepper, to taste

1. Put the cucumber, mint, yogurt, and garlic in a food processor, then pulse until creamy and smooth.
2. Transfer the puréed mixture in a large serving bowl, then add the vegetable soup, tomato paste, dill, salt, and ground black pepper. Stir to mix well.
3. Keep the soup in the refrigerator for at least 2 hours, then serve chilled.

Per Serving

calories: 133 | fat: 1.5g | protein: 14.2g | carbs: 16.5g | fiber: 2.9g | sodium: 331mg

Veggie Slaw

Prep time: 20 minutes | Cook time: 0 minutes | Serves 4 to 6

Salad:

2 large broccoli stems, peeled and shredded

½ celery root bulb, peeled and shredded

¼ cup chopped fresh Italian parsley

1 large beet, peeled and shredded

2 carrots, peeled and shredded

1 small red onion, sliced thin

2 zucchinis, shredded

Dressing:

1 teaspoon Dijon mustard

½ cup apple cider vinegar

1 tablespoon raw honey

1 teaspoon sea salt

¼ teaspoon freshly ground black pepper

2 tablespoons extra-virgin olive oil

Topping:

½ cup crumbled feta cheese

1. Combine the ingredients for the salad in a large salad bowl, then toss to combine well.
2. Combine the ingredients for the dressing in a small bowl, then stir to mix well.

3. Dress the salad, then serve with feta cheese on top.

Per Serving

calories: 387 | fat: 30.2g | protein: 8.1g | carbs: 25.9g | fiber: 6.0g | sodium: 980mg

Moroccan Lentil, Tomato, and Cauliflower Soup

Prep time: 15 minutes | Cook time: 4 hours | Serves 6

1 cup chopped carrots

1 cup chopped onions

3 cloves garlic, minced

½ teaspoon ground coriander

1 teaspoon ground cumin

1 teaspoon ground turmeric

¼ teaspoon ground cinnamon

¼ teaspoon freshly ground black pepper

1 cup dry lentils

28 ounces (794 g) tomatoes, diced, reserve the juice

1½ cups chopped cauliflower

4 cups low-sodium vegetable soup

1 tablespoon no-salt-added tomato paste

1 teaspoon extra-virgin olive oil

1 cup chopped fresh spinach

¼ cup chopped fresh cilantro

1 tablespoon red wine vinegar (optional)

1. Put the carrots and onions in the slow cooker, then sprinkle with minced garlic, coriander, cumin, turmeric, cinnamon, and black pepper. Stir to combine well.

2. Add the lentils, tomatoes, and cauliflower, then pour in the vegetable soup and tomato paste. Drizzle with olive oil. Stir to combine well.
3. Put the slow cooker lid on and cook on high for 4 hours or until the vegetables are tender.
4. In the last 30 minutes during the cooking time, open the lid and stir the soup, then fold in the spinach.
5. Pour the cooked soup in a large serving bowl, then spread with cilantro and drizzle with vinegar. Serve immediately.

Per Serving

calories: 131 | fat: 2.1g | protein: 5.6g | carbs: 25.0g | fiber: 5.5g | sodium: 364mg

Mushroom and Soba Noodle Soup

Prep time: 15 minutes | Cook time: 10 minutes | Serves 4

2 tablespoons coconut oil

8 ounces (227 g) shiitake mushrooms, stemmed and sliced thin

1 tablespoon minced fresh ginger

4 scallions, sliced thin

1 garlic clove, minced

1 teaspoon sea salt

4 cups low-sodium vegetable broth

3 cups water

4 ounces (113 g) soba noodles

1 bunch spinach, blanched, rinsed and cut into strips

1 tablespoon freshly squeezed lemon juice

1. Heat the coconut oil in a stockpot over medium heat until melted.
2. Add the mushrooms, ginger, scallions, garlic, and salt. Sauté for 5 minutes or until fragrant and the mushrooms are tender.
3. Pour in the vegetable broth and water. Bring to a boil, then add the soba noodles and cook for 5 minutes or until al dente.

4. Turn off the heat and add the spinach and lemon juice. Stir to mix well.
5. Pour the soup in a large bowl and serve immediately.

Per Serving

calories: 254 | fat: 9.2g | protein: 13.1g | carbs: 33.9g | fiber: 4.0g | sodium: 1773mg

Sandwiches, Pizzas, and Wraps

Alfalfa Sprout and Nut Rolls

Prep time: 40 minutes | Cook time: 0 minutes | Makes 16 bite-size pieces

1 cup alfalfa sprouts

2 tablespoons Brazil nuts

½ cup chopped fresh cilantro

2 tablespoons flaked coconut

1 garlic clove, minced

2 tablespoons ground flaxseeds

Zest and juice of 1 lemon

Pinch cayenne pepper

Sea salt and freshly ground black pepper, to taste

1 tablespoon melted coconut oil

2 tablespoons water

2 whole-grain wraps

1. Combine all ingredients, except for the wraps, in a food processor, then pulse to combine well until smooth.
2. Unfold the wraps on a clean work surface, then spread the mixture over the wraps. Roll the

wraps up and refrigerate for 30 minutes until set.

3. Remove the rolls from the refrigerator and slice into 16 bite-sized pieces, if desired, and serve.

Per Serving (1 piece)

calories: 67 | fat: 7.1g | protein: 2.2g | carbs: 2.9g | fiber: 1.0g | sodium: 61mg

Mini Pork and Cucumber Lettuce Wraps

Prep time: 20 minutes | Cook time: 0 minutes | Makes 12 wraps

8 ounces (227 g) cooked ground pork

1 cucumber, diced

1 tomato, diced

1 red onion, sliced

1 ounce (28 g) low-fat feta cheese, crumbled

Juice of 1 lemon

1 tablespoon extra-virgin olive oil

Sea salt and freshly ground pepper, to taste

12 small, intact iceberg lettuce leaves

1. Combine the ground pork, cucumber, tomato, and onion in a large bowl, then scatter with feta cheese. Drizzle with lemon juice and olive oil, and sprinkle with salt and pepper. Toss to mix well.
2. Unfold the small lettuce leaves on a large plate or several small plates, then divide and top with the pork mixture.
3. Wrap and serve immediately.

Per Serving (1 warp)

calories: 78 | fat: 5.6g | protein: 5.5g | carbs: 1.4g | fiber: 0.3g | sodium: 50mg

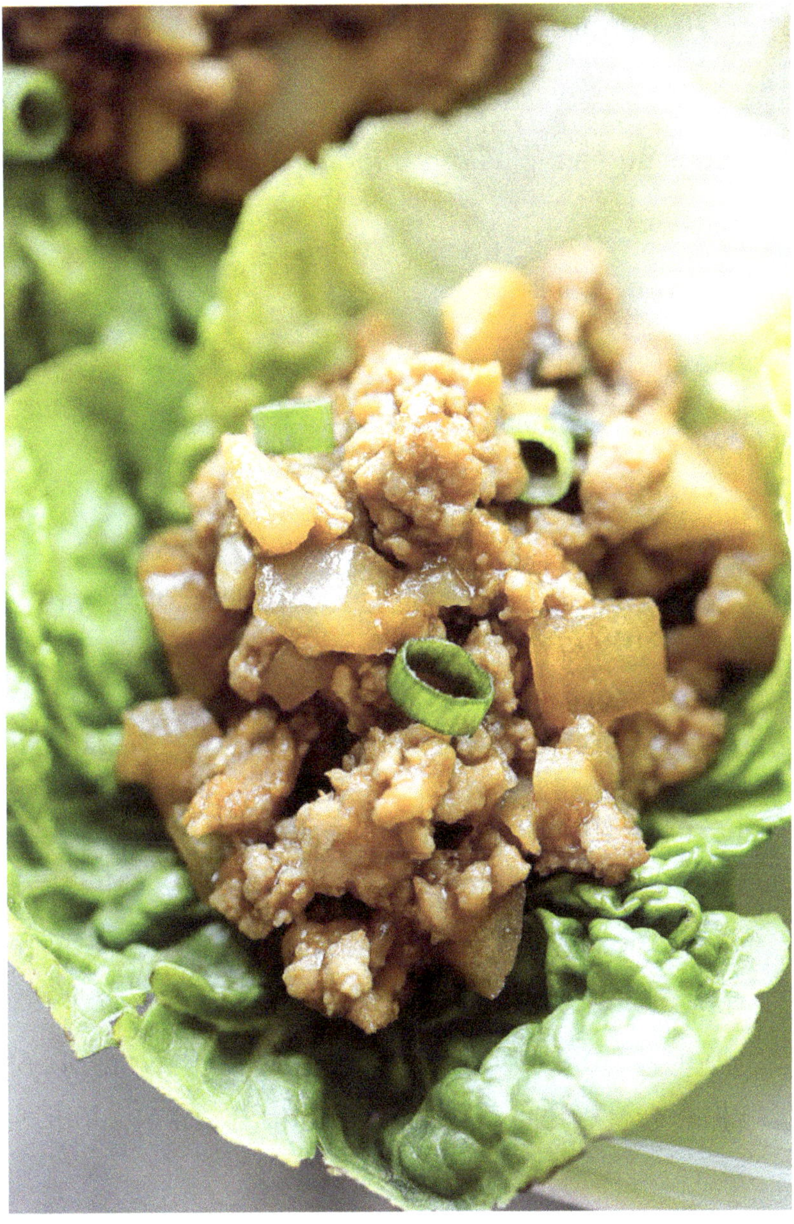

Mushroom and Caramelized Onion Musakhan

Prep time: 20 minutes | Cook time: 1 hour 5 minutes | Serves 4

2 tablespoons sumac, plus more for sprinkling

1 teaspoon ground allspice

½ teaspoon ground cardamom

½ teaspoon ground cumin

3 tablespoons extra-virgin olive oil, divided

2 pounds (907 g) portobello mushroom caps, gills removed, caps halved and sliced ½ inch thick

3 medium white onions, coarsely chopped

¼ cup water

Kosher salt, to taste

1 whole-wheat Turkish flatbread

¼ cup pine nuts

1 lemon, wedged

1. Preheat the oven to 350ºF (180ºC).
2. Combine 2 tablespoons of sumac, allspice, cardamom, and cumin in a small bowl. Stir to mix well.
3. Heat 2 tablespoons of olive oil in an oven-proof skillet over medium-high heat until shimmering.

4. Add the mushroom to the skillet and sprinkle with half of sumac mixture. Sauté for 8 minutes or until the mushrooms are tender. You may need to work in batches to avoid overcrowding. Transfer the mushrooms to a plate and set side.
5. Heat 1 tablespoon of olive oil in the skillet over medium-high heat until shimmering.
6. Add the onion and sauté for 20 minutes or until caramelized. Sprinkle with remaining sumac mixture, then cook for 1 more minute.
7. Pour in the water and sprinkle with salt. Bring to a simmer.
8. Turn off the heat and put the mushroom back to the skillet.
9. Place the skillet in the preheated oven and bake for 30 minutes.
10. Remove the skillet from the oven and let the mushroom sit for 10 minutes until cooled down.
11. Heat the Turkish flatbread in a baking dish in the oven for 5 minutes or until warmed through.
12. Arrange the bread on a large plate and top with mushrooms, onions, and roasted pine

nuts. Squeeze the lemon wedges over and sprinkle with more sumac. Serve immediately.

Per Serving

calories: 336 | fat: 18.7g | protein: 11.5g | carbs: 34.3g | fiber: 6.9g | sodium: 369mg

Red Pepper Coques with Pine Nuts

Prep time: 1 day 40 minutes | Cook time: 45 minutes | Makes 4 coques

Dough:

3 cups almond flour

½ teaspoon instant or rapid-rise yeast

2 teaspoons raw honey

1⅓ cups ice water

3 tablespoons extra-virgin olive oil

1½ teaspoons sea salt

Red Pepper Topping:

4 tablespoons extra-virgin olive oil, divided

2 cups jarred roasted red peppers, patted dry and sliced thinly

2 large onions, halved and sliced thin

3 garlic cloves, minced

¼ teaspoon red pepper flakes

2 bay leaves

3 tablespoons maple syrup

1½ teaspoons sea salt

3 tablespoons red whine vinegar

For Garnish:

¼ cup pine nuts (optional)

1 tablespoon minced fresh parsley

Make the Dough

1. Combine the flour, yeast, and honey in a food processor, pulse to combine well. Gently add water while pulsing. Let the dough sit for 10 minutes.
2. Mix the olive oil and salt in the dough and knead the dough until smooth. Wrap in plastic and refrigerate for at least 1 day.

Make the Topping

3. Heat 1 tablespoon of olive oil in a nonstick skillet over medium heat until shimmering.
4. Add the red peppers, onions, garlic, red pepper flakes, bay leaves, maple syrup, and salt. Sauté for 20 minutes or until the onion is caramelized.
5. Turn off the heat and discard the bay leaves. Remove the onion from the skillet and baste with wine vinegar. Let them sit until ready to use.

Make the Coques

6. Preheat the oven to 500ºF (260ºC). Grease two baking sheets with 1 tablespoon of olive oil.
7. Divide the dough ball into four balls, then press and shape them into equal-sized oval. Arrange

the ovals on the baking sheets and pierce each dough about 12 times.

8. Rub the ovals with 2 tablespoons of olive oil and bake for 7 minutes or until puffed. Flip the ovals halfway through the cooking time.
9. Spread the ovals with the topping and pine nuts, then bake for an additional 15 minutes or until well browned.
10. Remove the coques from the oven and spread with parsley. Allow to cool for 10 minutes before serving.

Per Serving (1 coque)

calories: 658 | fat: 23.1g | protein: 3.4g | carbs: 112.0g | fiber: 6.2g | sodium: 1757mg

Ritzy Garden Burgers

Prep time: 1 hour 30 minutes | Cook time: 30 minutes | Serves 6

- 1 tablespoon avocado oil
- 1 yellow onion, diced
- ½ cup shredded carrots
- 4 garlic cloves, halved
- 1 (15 ounces / 425 g) can black beans, rinsed and drained
- 1 cup gluten-free rolled oats
- ¼ cup oil-packed sun-dried tomatoes, drained and chopped
- ½ cup sunflower seeds, toasted
- 1 teaspoon chili powder
- 1 teaspoon paprika
- 1 teaspoon ground cumin
- ¼ teaspoon ground red pepper flakes
- ¾ teaspoon sea salt
- ¼ teaspoon ground black pepper
- ¼ cup olive oil

For Serving:

- 6 whole-wheat buns, split in half and toasted
- 2 ripe avocados, sliced
- 1 cup kaiware sprouts or mung bean sprouts
- 1 ripe tomato, sliced

½ cup fresh parsley, stems removed

1. Line a baking sheet with parchment paper.
2. Heat 1 tablespoon of avocado oil in a nonstick skillet over medium heat.
3. Add the onion and carrots and sauté for 10 minutes or until the onion is caramelized.
4. Add the garlic and sauté for 30 seconds or until fragrant.
5. Transfer them into a food processor, then add the remaining ingredients, except for the olive oil. Pulse until chopped fine and the mixture holds together. Make sure not to purée the mixture.
6. Divide and form the mixture into six 4-inch diameter and ½-inch thick patties.
7. Arrange the patties on the baking sheet and wrap the sheet in plastic. Put the baking sheet in the refrigerator and freeze for at least an hour until firm.
8. Remove the baking sheet from the refrigerator, let them sit under room temperature for 10 minutes.

9. Heat the olive oil in a nonstick skillet over medium-high heat until shimmering.
10. Fry the patties in the skillet for 15 minutes or until lightly browned and crispy. Flip the patties halfway through the cooking time. You may need to work in batches to avoid overcrowding.
11. Assemble the buns with patties, avocados, sprouts, and tomato slices to make the burgers.

Per Serving

calories: 613 | fat: 23.1g | protein: 26.2g | carbs: 88.3g | fiber: 22.9g | sodium: 456mg

Roasted Tomato Panini

Prep time: 15 minutes | Cook time: 3 hours 6 minutes | Serves 2

2 teaspoons olive oil

4 Roma tomatoes, halved

4 cloves garlic

1 tablespoon Italian seasoning

Sea salt and freshly ground pepper, to taste

4 slices whole-grain bread

4 basil leaves

2 slices fresh Mozzarella cheese

1. Preheat the oven to 250ºF (121ºC). Grease a baking pan with olive oil.
2. Place the tomatoes and garlic in the baking pan, then sprinkle with Italian seasoning, salt, and ground pepper. Toss to coat well.
3. Roast in the preheated oven for 3 hours or until the tomatoes are lightly wilted.
4. Preheat the panini press.
5. Make the panini: Place two slices of bread on a clean work surface, then top them with wilted tomatoes. Sprinkle with basil and spread with Mozzarella cheese. Top them with remaining two slices of bread.

6. Cook the panini for 6 minutes or until lightly browned and the cheese melts. Flip the panini halfway through the cooking.
7. Serve immediately.

Per Serving

calories: 323 | fat: 12.0g | protein: 17.4g | carbs: 37.5g | fiber: 7.5g | sodium: 603mg

Samosas in Potatoes

Prep time: 20 minutes | Cook time: 30 minutes | Makes 8

4 small potatoes

1 teaspoon coconut oil

1 small onion, finely chopped

1 small piece ginger, minced

2 garlic cloves, minced

2 to 3 teaspoons curry powder

Sea salt and freshly ground black pepper, to taste

¼ cup frozen peas, thawed

2 carrots, grated

¼ cup chopped fresh cilantro

1. Preheat the oven to 350ºF (180ºC).
2. Poke small holes into potatoes with a fork, then wrap with aluminum foil.
3. Bake in the preheated oven for 30 minutes until tender.
4. Meanwhile, heat the coconut oil in a nonstick skillet over medium-high heat until melted.
5. Add the onion and sauté for 5 minutes or until translucent.

6. Add the ginger and garlic to the skillet and sauté for 3 minutes or until fragrant.
7. Add the curry powder, salt, and ground black pepper, then stir to coat the onion. Remove them from the heat.
8. When the cooking of potatoes is complete, remove the potatoes from the foil and slice in half.
9. Hollow to potato halves with a spoon, then combine the potato fresh with sautéed onion, peas, carrots, and cilantro in a large bowl. Stir to mix well.
10. Spoon the mixture back to the tomato skins and serve immediately.

Per Serving (1 samosa)

calories: 131 | fat: 13.9g | protein: 3.2g | carbs: 8.8g | fiber: 3.0g | sodium: 111mg

Spicy Black Bean and Poblano Dippers

Prep time: 20 minutes | Cook time: 21 minutes | Serves 8

2 tablespoons avocado oil, plus more for brushing the dippers

1 (15 ounces / 425 g) can black beans, drained and rinsed

1 poblano, deseeded and quartered

1 jalapeño, halved and deseeded

½ cup fresh cilantro, leaves and tender stems

1 yellow onion, quartered

2 garlic cloves

1 teaspoon chili powder

1 teaspoon ground cumin

1 teaspoon sea salt

24 organic corn tortillas

1. Preheat the oven to 400ºF (205ºC). Line a baking sheet with parchment paper and grease with avocado oil.
2. Combine the remaining ingredients, except for the tortillas, in a food processor, then pulse until chopped finely and the mixture holds together. Make sure not to purée the mixture.

3. Warm the tortillas on the baking sheet in the preheated oven for 1 minute or until softened.
4. Add a tablespoon of the mixture in the middle of each tortilla. Fold one side of the tortillas over the mixture and tuck to roll them up tightly to make the dippers.
5. Arrange the dippers on the baking sheet and brush them with avocado oil.
1. Bake in the oven for 20 minutes or until well browned. Flip the dippers halfway through the cooking time.
6. Serve immediately.

Per Serving

calories: 388 | fat: 6.5g | protein: 16.2g | carbs: 69.6g | fiber: 13.5g | sodium: 340mg

Spicy Tofu Tacos with Cherry Tomato Salsa

Prep time: 20 minutes | Cook time: 11 minutes | Makes 4 tacos

Cherry Tomato Salsa:

¼ cup sliced cherry tomatoes

½ jalapeño, deseeded and sliced

Juice of 1 lime

1 garlic clove, minced

Sea salt and freshly ground black pepper, to taste

2 teaspoons extra-virgin olive oil

Spicy Tofu Taco Filling:

4 tablespoons water, divided

½ cup canned black beans, rinsed and drained

2 teaspoons fresh chopped chives, divided

¾ teaspoon ground cumin, divided

¾ teaspoon smoked paprika, divided

Dash cayenne pepper (optional)

¼ teaspoon sea salt

¼ teaspoon freshly ground black pepper

1 teaspoon extra-virgin olive oil

6 ounces (170 g) firm tofu, drained, rinsed, and pressed

4 corn tortillas

¼ avocado, sliced

¼ cup fresh cilantro

Make the Cherry Tomato Salsa

1. Combine the ingredients for the salsa in a small bowl. Stir to mix well. Set aside until ready to use.

Make the Spicy Tofu Taco Filling

2. Add 2 tablespoons of water into a saucepan, then add the black beans and sprinkle with 1 teaspoon of chives, ½ teaspoon of cumin, ¼ teaspoon of smoked paprika, and cayenne. Stir to mix well.
3. Cook for 5 minutes over medium heat until heated through, then mash the black beans with the back of a spoon. Turn off the heat and set aside.
4. Add remaining water into a bowl, then add the remaining chives, cumin, and paprika. Sprinkle with cayenne, salt, and black pepper. Stir to mix well. Set aside.
5. Heat the olive oil in a nonstick skillet over medium heat until shimmering.
6. Add the tofu and drizzle with taco sauce, then sauté for 5 minutes or until the seasoning is

absorbed. Remove the tofu from the skillet and set aside.

7. Warm the tortillas in the skillet for 1 minutes or until heated through.
8. Transfer the tortillas onto a large plate and top with tofu, mashed black beans, avocado, cilantro, then drizzle the tomato salsa over. Serve immediately.

Per Serving (1 taco)

calories: 240 | fat: 9.0g | protein: 11.6g | carbs: 31.6g | fiber: 6.7g | sodium: 195mg

Super Cheeses and Mushroom Tart

Prep time: 30 minutes | Cook time: 1 hour 30 minutes | Serves 4 to 6

Crust:

1¾ cups almond flour

1 tablespoon raw honey

¾ teaspoon sea salt

¼ cup extra-virgin olive oil

⅓ cup water

Filling:

2 tablespoons extra-virgin olive oil, divided

1 pound (454 g) white mushrooms, trimmed and sliced thinly

Sea salt, to taste

1 garlic clove, minced

2 teaspoons minced fresh thyme

¼ cup shredded Mozzarella cheese

½ cup grated Parmesan cheese

4 ounces (113 g) part-skim ricotta cheese

Ground black pepper, to taste

2 tablespoons ground basil

Make the Crust

1. Preheat the oven to 350ºF (180ºC).

2. Combine the flour, honey, salt and olive oil in a large bowl. Stir to mix well. Gently mix in the water until a smooth dough forms.
3. Drop walnut-size clumps from the dough in the single layer on a tart pan. Press the clumps to coat the bottom of the pan.
4. Bake the crust in the preheated oven for 50 minutes or until firm and browned. Rotate the pan halfway through.

Make the Filling

5. While baking the crust, heat 1 tablespoon of olive oil in a nonstick skillet over medium-high heat until shimmering.
6. Add the mushrooms and sprinkle with ½ teaspoon of salt. Sauté for 15 minutes or until tender.
7. Add the garlic and thyme and sauté for 30 seconds or until fragrant.

Make the Tart

8. Meanwhile, combine the cheeses, salt, ground black pepper, and 1 tablespoon of olive oil in a bowl. Stir to mix well.
9. Spread the cheese mixture over the crust, then top with the mushroom mixture.

10. Bake in the oven for 20 minutes or until the cheeses are frothy and the tart is heated through. Rotate the pan halfway through the baking time.
11. Remove the tart from the oven. Allow to cool for at least 10 minutes, then sprinkle with basil. Slice to serve.

Per Serving

calories: 530 | fat: 26.6g | protein: 11.7g | carbs: 63.5g | fiber: 4.6g | sodium: 785mg

CPSIA information can be obtained
at www.ICGtesting.com
Printed in the USA
BVHW091128210621
610125BV00004B/876

9 781803 177243